Healthy Pressure Cooker Recipes Cookbook

Flavorful Pressure Cooker Recipes for Any Taste and Occasion

Ruth P. Baldwin

Sommario

Introduction

Vegetarianism describes a way of life that leaves out the intake of all kinds of meat, including pork, hen, beef, lamb, venison, fish, and also shells.
Relying on an individual's beliefs and way of living, vegetarianism has various ranges. There are vegetarians who like to eat products that originate from animals such as milk, eggs, lotion as well as cheese. At the various other end of the range are vegans.
Vegans never consume meat or any type of products that come from pets.

The vegan diet has many benefits, actually, the non-meat intake even adhering to the viewpoint of numerous professionals can likewise be a benefit for our body.

Actually, this type of diet plan is an exceptional means to attain peace between your body and your mind, constantly keep in mind not to desert your concepts.

Enjoy reading our delicious dishes.

healthy dishes

Pasta Soup with Veg

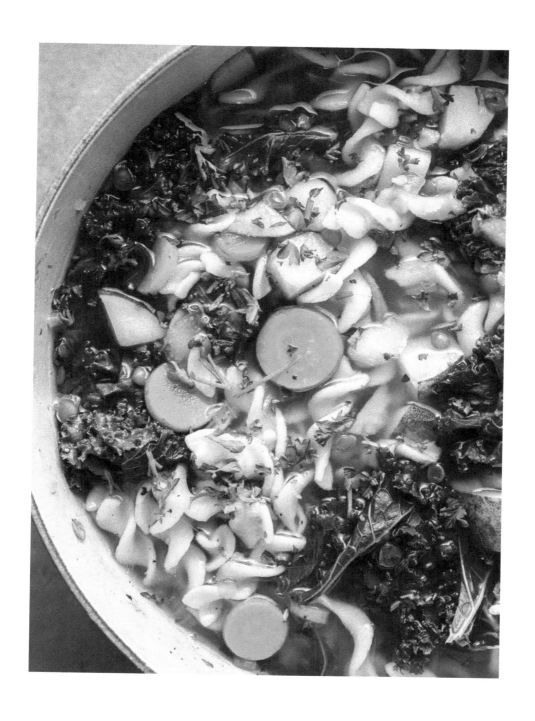

Ingredients for 6 serving:

2 stalks celery diced 1 large carrot diced 1 small yellow onion

diced 1 small red bell pepper diced 2 teaspoons dried parsley 1 bay leaf 6 cups vegetable broth 28 ounce kidney beans rinsed and drained, 2 cans 1 ½ cups pasta dry 3 cups baby spinach fresh 1 cup mushrooms sliced ⅛ teaspoon black pepper ground

Directions and total time – 30-60 m

• Press the "Sauté" button; add celery, carrot, onion, bell pepper, dried parsley, bay leaf and ¼ cup vegetable broth. • Sauté vegetables in broth until onions are translucent, about 8 minutes. If the inner pot becomes dry before onion is tender, add 2 tablespoons broth to prevent vegetables from sticking. • Add remaining broth, kidney beans, pasta, spinach, mushrooms, and pepper. • Continue to simmer soup until pasta is tender to the bite, 10 to 15 minutes, depending on pasta type. • Remove bay leaf. Press "Keep Warm/Cancel" twice to activate keep warm mode. • Serve right away or cover with lid, the soup is ready when your family is ready to eat.

Soup White Bean and Kale

Ingredients for 6 servings:

1 lb dried white beans 2 stalks celery chopped 1 medium yellow onion peeled and diced 1 garlic clove minced 3 cups chopped kale 1 tsp salt ½ tsp black pepper 6 cups vegetable broth 1 tbsp olive oil

Directions and total time – 30-60 m

• In a large bowl, soak beans overnight in water to cover. Drain and add to the Instant Pot. • Add remaining ingredients to the Instant Pot. Close lid, set steam release to Sealing, press the Manual button, and adjust time to 20 minutes. When the timer beeps, let pressure release naturally, about 20 minutes. • Remove lid and stir well. Serve hot.

Minestrone Soup with Beans

Ingredients for 4 servings:

2 cups dried great Northern beans 1 cup orzo 2 large carrots peeled and diced 1 bunch Swiss chard ribs removed and roughly chopped 1 medium zucchini diced 2 stalks celery diced 1 medium onion peeled and diced 1 tsp minced Garlic 1 tbsp Italian seasoning 1 tsp salt ½ tsp ground black pepper 2 bay leaves 14 ½ oz diced tomatoes including juice (1 can) 4 cups vegetable broth 1 cup tomato juice 4 sprigs fresh parsley for garnish

Directions and total time – 30-60 m

● Rinse beans and add to the Instant Pot with remaining ingredients except parsley. Lock the lid. ● Press the Soup button and cook for the default time of 30 minutes. ● When timer beeps, let pressure release naturally for 10 minutes. ● Quick-release any additional pressure until float valve drops and then unlock lid. Ladle

14

into bowls, garnish each bowl with a sprig of parsley, and serve warm.

Smoked White Beans and Sausage

Ingredients for 6 servings:

2 tsp olive oil 1 lb smoked sausage cut into ½ inch disks, pork or turkey 1 small onion finely chopped 2 carrots diced 2 celery stalks diced 4 cups chicken broth (low-sodium), warmed 1 lb dried small white beans rinsed and picked over, like navy beans 1 tbsp chopped fresh thyme OR 1 tbsp cajun seasoning

Directions and total time – 1-2 h

• Add olive oil to the Instant Pot. Using the display panel select the SAUTE function. • When oil gets hot, brown the cut sausage on both sides. Transfer browned meat to a shallow dish and cover loosely with foil. • Add onion, carrots and celery to the pot and saute until onion is soft, 3-4 minutes. • Add broth to the pot and deglaze by using a wooden spoon to scrape the brown bits from the bottom of the pot. • Put the sausage back into the pot, add sorted and rinsed beans and stir to combine. • Turn the pot off by selecting CANCEL, then secure the lid, making sure the vent is closed. • Using the display panel select the MANUAL function. Use the +/-keys and program the Instant Pot for 60 minutes. • When the time is up, let the pressure naturally release for 15 minutes, then quick-release the remaining pressure. • Serve hot, alongside fresh cornbread (optional).

Black Beans, Quinoa and Corn

Ingredients for 6 servings:

1 tablespoon ground chipotle powder 2 teaspoons ground cumin 2 tablespoons dried onion 1 teaspoon dried garlic 1 teaspoon Mexican oregano 2 cups quick-cooking quinoa 1 cup dehydrated black beans ½ cup dried corn 4 cups vegetable broth or water roughly chopped fresh cilantro to serve lime juice to serve

Directions and total time – 15 m

• Layer the dry ingredients in the jar in the order listed. • Place all of the jarred ingredients into the Instant Pot. Add 4 cups of broth or water. Stir to mix. Cover with the lid and ensure the vent is in the "Sealed" position. Pressure Cook on High for 5 minutes. Allow the steam pressure to release naturally for 5 minutes, then release any remaining pressure manually. To Serve: • Garnish with fresh cilantro and a squeeze of lime juice.

Greek-Style Gigantes Beans with Feta

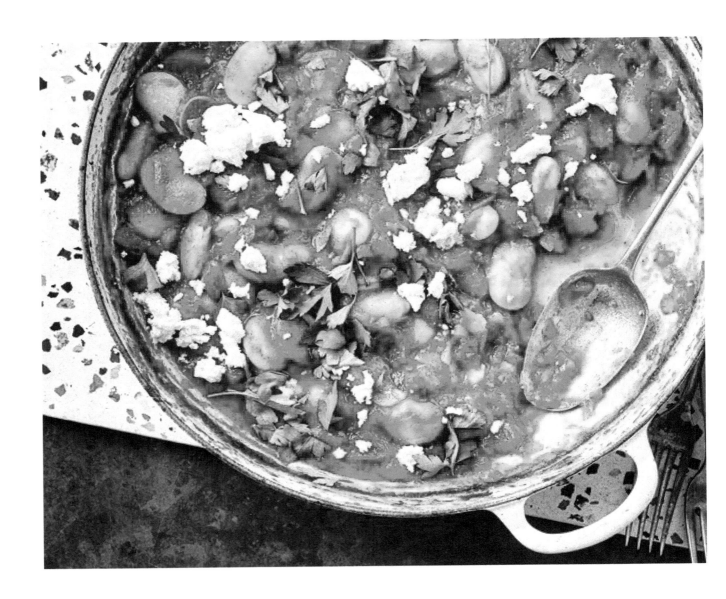

Ingredients for 8 servings:

3 cups dried gigantes or other large white beans like lima beans 8 cups Water 1 ½ teaspoons kosher salt ¼ cup extra-virgin olive oil plus 2 additional tablespoons 1 clove garlic peeled 1 large yellow onion finely diced 1 stalk celery finely diced 28 ounces crushed tomatoes about 3 cups, 1 can 1 teaspoon dried oregano ¼ teaspoon black pepper freshly ground ¼ cup flat-leaf parsley chopped fresh ½ cup feta cheese crumbled

Directions and total time – 30 m

• Combine the beans, water, and salt in the Instant Pot. Leave the pot turned off and let the beans soak for 10 to 12 hours or up to overnight. • Secure the lid and set the Pressure Release to Sealing. Select the Bean/Chili setting and set the cooking time for 15 minutes at high pressure. • Let the pressure release naturally for 15 minutes, then move the Pressure Release to Venting to release any remaining steam. Open the pot, ladle out 1 cup of the cooking liquid, and set the liquid aside. Wearing heat-resistant mitts, lift the inner pot out of the Instant Pot and drain the beans in a colander. Return the now-empty inner pot to the Instant Pot housing. • Select the Sauté setting and heat the ¼ cup olive oil in the pot. Add the garlic, onion, and celery and sauté for about 5 minutes, until the onion has softened. Add the drained beans, the reserved 1 cup liquid, the tomatoes, oregano, and pepper and stir well. • Secure the lid and set the Pressure Release to Sealing. Press the Cancel button to reset the cooking program, then select the Bean/Chili setting and set the cooking time for 5 minutes at high pressure. • Let the pressure release naturally for at least 15 minutes, then move the Pressure Release to Venting to release any remaining steam. • Ladle the beans into a serving dish. Sprinkle the parsley and feta cheese over the beans, drizzle with the remaining 2 tablespoons olive oil, and serve.

Soup with Ham and Pinto Bean

Ingredients for 4-6 servings:

1 ½ - 2 lbs smoked pork hocks rinsed 1 cup diced ham 1 small onion finely diced 6 cloves of garlic minced 1 tsp celery seed (or 2 ribs celery diced) 1 tsp ground cumin ¼ tsp dried oregano 2 bay leaves 1 lb dried pinto beans rinsed (you do not need to soak) 3 cups unsalted chicken stock 2 cups Water salt and pepper to taste ¼ cup diced cilantro ½ cup diced fresh tomatoes

Directions and total time – 1-2 h

• Add all ingredients except the Toppings to the Instant Pot, then secure the lid, making sure the vent is closed. • Using the display panel select the MANUAL or PRESSURE COOK function. Use the +/- keys and program the Instant Pot for 50 minutes. • When the time is up, let the pressure naturally release for 20 minutes, then quick-release the remaining pressure. • Remove pork hock, slice any remaining meat from the bone and return to the pot. • Serve warm topped with cilantro and tomatoes alongside cornbread or biscuits.

Black Beans with Apple, Chicken and Sausage

Ingredients for 4-6 servings:

1 ½ tbsp olive oil 12 ounces package chicken & apple sausage sliced into ⅓" disks 30 ounces ranch Style black beans not drained, 2 cans 15 ounces 1 ½ tsp onion salt eachand 1 ½ tsp onion powder ⅓ cup brown sugar ¼ cup sour cream 1 tbsp chives snipped

Directions and total time – 15-30 m

• Add olive oil to the Instant Pot. Using the display panel select the SAUTE function. • When oil is hot, add sliced sausage, Cook and stir 3-4 minutes until lightly browned. • Add beans, onion salt, onion powder and brown sugar. • Using the display panel select the MANUAL or PRESSURE COOK function. Use the +/- buttons and program the Instant Pot for 0 (zero) minutes. • When the time is up, quick-release the remaining pressure. • Serve topped with a dollop of sour cream and a dusting of chives.

Andouille with Red Beans and Rice

Ingredients for 6 servings:

1 cup uncooked white rice ½ teaspoon salt chopped parsley for garnish 1 cup dried red beans 1 pound cooked andouille sausage sliced 2 stalks celery sliced 1 medium green bell pepper seeded and diced ½ medium onion diced 1 clove garlic minced 1 teaspoon dried oregano 1 teaspoon salt ½ teaspoon cayenne pepper

Directions and total time – 1-2 h Prepare Rice:

• Add the rice, salt, and 1 ½ cups water to the Instant Pot inner pot and stir. Secure the lid, ensuring the valve is turned to the Sealing position. Select the Rice button. The timer will selfcalculate. • Once cooking is complete, turn the valve to the Venting position to release the pressure. When all the pressure is released, carefully remove the lid. Fluff the rice with a fork. Transfer the rice to a large bowl, garnish with parsley, and set aside. Wash and dry the inner pot. • Add all the remaining ingredients plus 3 cups water to the inner pot and stir well. Secure the lid, ensuring the valve is turned to the Sealing position. Press the Pressure Cook button and set the time to 45 minutes. • Once cooking is complete, allow the appliance to natural release for 10 minutes. After 10 minutes, turn the valve to the Venting position to release the pressure. • When all the pressure is released, carefully remove the lid and stir well. Serve the bean/ sausage mixture and rice either separately or combined.

Soup Cannellini Beans and Kale

Ingredients for 6 servings:

2 tablespoons olive oil plus more for garnish ¼ cup pancetta diced, from a ½-inch- thick slab, or chopped thick-cut bacon 1 medium yellow onion chopped 1 carrot finely diced 1 rib celery finely diced 3 cloves garlic chopped 4 cups savoy cabbage chopped 4 cups lacinato kale chopped, including center ribs 4 cups vegetable broth or chicken, homemade or low-sodium store-bought 3 cups cannellini beans soaked, from 1 ½ cups dried beans 1 rind Parmesan cheese 2-inch, optional 1 pinch red chile flakes Salt and pepper 2 cups rustic bread 1-inch pieces, crusts discarded, 4 ounces ½ cup marinara sauce homemade or jarred, warmed

Directions and total time – 1-2 h

● Put the oil in the pot, select Saute, and adjust to More/High heat. When the oil is hot, add the pancetta and cook, stirring occasionally, until it begins to brown, 2 minutes. Carefully spoon out all but 1 tablespoon of the fat. • Add the onion, carrot, and celery to the pot and cook, stirring, until the onion is just tender, 4 minutes. Add the garlic and cook until fragrant, 45 seconds. Press Cancel. • Add the cabbage, kale, broth, beans, cheese rind (if using), red chili flakes, ½ teaspoon salt, and several grinds of pepper. Lock on the lid, select the Pressure Cook function, and adjust to High pressure for 15 minutes. Make sure the steam valve is in the "Sealing" position and that the "Keep Warm" button is off. • When the cooking time is up, let the pressure come down naturally for 10 minutes and then quick- release the remaining pressure. Stir the bread and marinara sauce into the soup and let stand for 2 minutes. Discard the cheese rind and season the soup with salt and pepper. • Ladle the soup into bowls and garnish with a drizzle of olive oil, if desired.

Romano Beans Purple Yam with Barley

Ingredients for 12 servings:

3 tablespoons pearl barley 3 tablespoons pot barley 3 tablespoons buckwheat 3 tablespoons glutinous rice 3 tablespoons black glutinous rice 3 tablespoons black eye beans 3 tablespoons red beans 3 tablespoons romano beans 3 tablespoons brown rice 1 purple yam about 10.5 ounces ⅙ teaspoon baking soda optional

Directions and total time – 30-60 m

• Clean the purple yam, remove the skin and cut into 1 centimetre cubes. • Wash the barley, rice and beans in the inner pot of Instant Pot. • Place the purple yam and baking soda (if using) into the pot. • Add water up to the 8 cup mark on the inner pot. • Close the lid and put the steam release to the Sealing position. Select the [Porridge] program and keep pressing until the "More" setting is selected. • After the program finishes, let it cool for 10 minutes.

Don't try to release the pres- sure as the starchy porridge will spill

out. • Serve plain or with sugar, honey or blue agave syrup.

Beans Soup

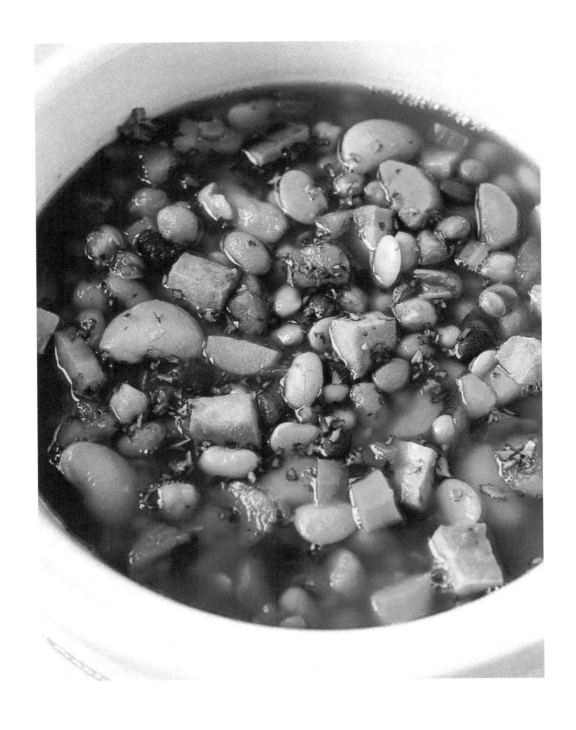

Ingredients for 4-6 servings:

½ cup yellow onion chopped 2 cloves garlic minced ½ cup Zucchini chopped ½ red bell pepper diced (about ½ cup) 1 cup green beans fresh, string removed and cut into thirds 1 cup Eggplant cut into cubes 1 stalk celery diced ½ cup carrot chopped 1 small russet potato diced ¼ cup parsley chopped 15.5 ounce garbanzo beans rinsed and drained well, 1 can. 12 ounce tomatoes diced, 1 can 2 teaspoons basil dried 2 teaspoons oregano 10 turns black pepper 1 teaspoon salt 3 cups Water

Directions and total time – 15-30 m

• Prep and measure out all of the ingredients first. This will make it super easy to throw together. • Press Sauté on your Instant Pot and let the inner pot heat up for 2 minutes. • Add all of the ingredients, except for the water and sauté for 5 minutes, stirring regularly so that nothing sticks to the bottom of the pot (onion, garlic, zucchini, bell pepper, green beans, eggplant, celery, potato, parsley, garbanzo beans, tomatoes, basil, oregano, black pepper and salt). Add just a splash of water if the veggies start to stick. • Turn off the Instant Pot, add the water and stir. Lock the lid into place, making sure the nozzle is in the sealing position. • Use the Manual setting and set the timer for 10 minutes. When time is up, use the natural release method. When all of the pressure is out of the Instant Pot, take off the lid and allow to cool.

Creamy Turkey Soup

Ingredients for 8 servings:

2 tablespoons unsalted butter 2 medium carrots peeled and chopped 2 stalks celery chopped 1 medium onion peeled and chopped 2 garlic cloves peeled and minced 1 tsp poultry seasoning 1 tsp salt ½ tsp ground black pepper 1 cup uncooked wild rice 1 bone-in turkey breast skin removed, 6 pounds 4 cups chicken stock ⅓ cup Water 2 tbsp cornstarch ½ cup heavy cream

Directions and total time – 30-60 m

• Press the Sauté button on the Instant Pot and melt butter. Add carrots, celery, and onion. Cook until vegetables are just tender, about 4–5 minutes, then add garlic, poultry seasoning, salt, pepper, and rice and cook until garlic is fragrant, about 1 minute. • Add turkey breast to pot and toss to coat. Press the Cancel button, add stock, close lid, set steam release to Sealing, press the Manual button, and set time to 45 minutes. • When the timer beeps, quick-release the pressure, open lid, and stir well. Press the Cancel button. Transfer turkey breast to a cutting board and allow to cool slightly, then shred meat, discarding bones. Return turkey to pot. • Press the Sauté button. Whisk together water and cornstarch and stir into pot. Bring to a boil, stirring constantly, until thickened, about 3–4 minutes. Press the Cancel button and stir in cream. Serve hot.

Taco Turkey on Lettuce Boats

Ingredients for 4 servings:

1 tbsp avocado oil 1 medium onion peeled and diced 2 large carrots peeled and diced 2 medium stalks celery ends removed and diced 2 cloves garlic minced 1 lb lean ground turkey 1 tsp chili powder 1 tsp paprika 1 tsp cumin ½ tsp salt ¼ tsp black pepper 1 cup chipotle salsa 12 large romaine leaves 1 medium avocado peeled, pitted, and sliced

Directions and total time – 30-60 m

• Press the Sauté button and add the oil. Allow the oil to heat 1 minute and then add the onion, carrots, celery, and garlic. Cook until softened, about 5 minutes. • Add the turkey and cook until browned, about 3 minutes. • Add the chili powder, paprika, cumin, salt, pepper, and salsa and stir to combine. Press the Cancel button. Secure the lid. • Press the Manual or Pressure Cook button and adjust the time to 15 minutes. • When the timer beeps, quick-release pressure until float valve drops and then unlock lid. ● To serve, spoon a portion of the taco meat into a romaine lettuce leaf and then top with sliced avocado.

Ma Shu Turkey

Ingredients for 6 servings:

7 ounces plum sauce 1 jar, divided ¼ cup orange juice (juice of 1 medium orange) ¼ cup finely chopped onion 1 tbsp minced fresh ginger ¼ tsp salt ¼ tsp ground cinnamon 1 lb boneless turkey breast cut into thin strips 6 flour tortillas (7-inch) 3 cups coleslaw mix

Directions and total time – 10 m

• Combine ⅓ cup plum sauce, orange juice, onion, ginger, salt and cinnamon in Instant Pot®; mix well. Add turkey, stir to coat. • Secure lid and move pressure release valve to Sealing position. Press Manual or Pressure Cook; cook at high pressure 4 minutes. • When cooking is complete, press Cancel and use quick release. • Press Sauté; cook 2 to 3 minutes or until sauce is reduced and thickens slightly. • Spread remaining jarred plum sauce over tortillas; top with turkey and coleslaw mix. Fold bottom edge of tortillas over filling; fold in sides and roll up to completely

enclose filling. Serve with remaining cooking sauce for dipping.

Taco Salad with Turkey

Ingredients for 4 servings:

1 tbsp olive oil 1 lb ground turkey ½ tsp salt ½ tsp pepper 16 oz tub refrigerated fresh salsa 15 oz pinto beans 1 can drained and rinsed 2 tbsp sour cream 1 head romaine lettuce cut into pieces 9 oz tortilla chips 1 bag 1 large avocado diced 1 cup grated cheddar or monterey jack

Directions and total time – 15-30 m

• Add olive oil to the Instant Pot. Using the display panel select the SAUTE function and adjust to HIGH or MORE. • When oil gets hot, add the turkey, salt and pepper and brown the meat until no pink remains. • Stir in half the salsa and the drained pinto beans. • Turn the pot off by selecting CANCEL, then secure the lid, making sure the vent is closed. • Using the display panel select the MANUAL or PRESSURE COOK function. Use the +/- keys and program the Instant Pot for 4 minutes. • When the time is up, let the pressure naturally release for 4 minutes, then quick-release the remaining pressure. • In a small bowl, combine the remaining salsa and sour cream. • Divide the lettuce, chips, turkey/bean mixture, avocado, cheese and olives (if using) among bowls. Serve with the salsa-sour cream dressing.

Turkey Breast and Stuffing

Ingredients for 4 servings:

2 lbs uncooked turkey breast 1 tsp salt 1 tsp pepper ¾ cup chicken broth 6 oz stuffing mix 1 box 10.5 oz cream of chicken soup 1 can 8 oz sour cream plain greek yogurt or mayonnaise 2 cups frozen green beans

Directions and total time – 30-60 m

• Cut turkey breast into 4 pieces such that no piece is more than 1 inch thick. Season with salt and pepper. • Add broth to the pot and arrange turkey in an even layer, then secure the lid, making sure the vent is closed. • Using the display panel select the MANUAL or PRESSURE COOK function. Use the +/- keys and program the Instant Pot for 7 minutes. • Meanwhile, in a medium bowl, gently fold together stuffing mix, cream of chicken soup and sour cream just until combined. Do not overmix. • When the time is up, quick-release the remaining pressure and check to see if the turkey is fully cooked. (If it is not, add 2 tbsp water, reseal the pot and select MANUAL or PRESSURE COOK for an additional 2 minutes, then quick-release again.) • Place frozen green beans in an even layer on the turkey--do not stir. Reseal the pot and select MANUAL or PRESSURE COOK for 2 minutes, then quick-release the pressure. • Place stuffing mixture in an even layer on the green beans--do not stir. Reseal the pot and select MANUAL or PRESSURE COOK for 4 minutes, then quick-release any pressure. (Since the stuffing absorbs liquids, you may not get a complete seal in this step--don't worry.) • Serve hot with a side of cranberry sauce.

Turkey Breast Braised Stuffed

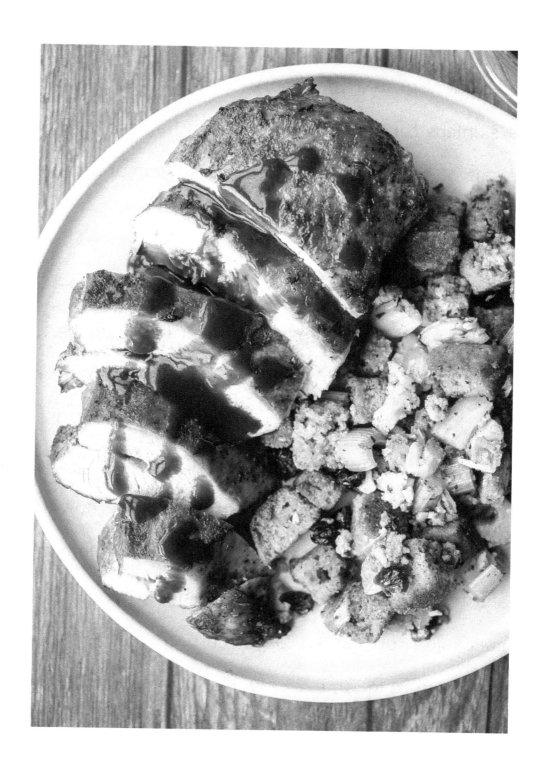

Ingredients for 4-6 servings: 2 tbsp butter 1 medium shallot minced 1 medium garlic clove peeled and minced (1 teaspoon) 4 ounces bulk sweet Italian sausage meat (or links with the casings removed) ¼ cup raisins chopped 1 cup fresh breadcrumbs 1 tsp lemon zest finely grated (optional) ½ tsp fennel seeds 2 ½ lbs boneless skinless turkey breast butterflied flat and opened up ½ tsp table salt ½ tsp ground black pepper 2 fresh oregano sprigs 1 ½ tbsp Water 1 tbsp cornstarch

Directions and total time – 30-60 m • Press Saute, set time for 10 minutes. • Melt 1 tablespoon butter in the cooker. Add the shallot and garlic; cook, stirring often, until softened, 2 minutes. Crumble in the sausage meat. Cook, stirring to break it up, until well browned, about 4 minutes. • Turn off the SAUTÉ function and scrape the contents of the pot's insert into a large bowl. Cool for 5 minutes; then stir in the raisins, breadcrumbs, lemon zest (if using), and fennel seeds. Cool for 10 minutes. • Lay the turkey breast split side up on a large cutting board. Spread the breadcrumb mixture in an even layer over the meat. Roll the meat up from the long edge to form a compact spiraled "log," then tie this log in three places with butchers' twine to keep it closed. Season the outside of the log with the salt and pepper. • Press Saute, set time for 10 minutes. • Melt the remaining 1 tablespoon butter in the cooker. Add the stuffed turkey breast (bending it to fit if need be) and brown lightly on all sides, turning occasionally, about 5 minutes. Turn off the SAUTÉ function, then pour in the broth. Tuck the oregano sprigs around the meat and lock the lid onto the cooker. • Optional 1 Max Pressure Cooker Press Pressure cook on Max pressure for 25 minutes with the Keep Warm setting off. • Optional 2 All Pressure Cookers Press Meat/Stew or Pressure cook (Manual) on High pressure for 35 minutes with the Keep Warm setting off. • When the machine has finished cooking, turn it off and let its pressure return to normal naturally, about 25 minutes. Unlatch the lid and open the cooker. Find and discard the oregano sprigs. Use a large, metal spatula and a spoon (for balance) to transfer the turkey roll to a nearby cutting board. • Press Saute, set time for 5 minutes. • As the sauce comes to a simmer, whisk the water and cornstarch in a small bowl until smooth. Whisk this slurry into the sauce and continue cooking, whisking constantly, until thickened somewhat,1 to 2 minutes. Immediately turn off the SAUTÉ function and remove the insert from the pot to stop the cooking. Slice the stuffed turkey breast into 1-inch-thick slices and serve with the sauce ladled on top.

Turkey Cheesy Soup

Ingredients for 8 servings: 1 pound ground turkey 2 teaspoons seasoned salt 1 tablespoon butter 2 carrots, diced 2 stalks celery, diced 1 medium onion, diced 2 tablespoons all-purpose flour 1 teaspoon dried dill weed ½ teaspoon ground black pepper 3 ½ cups beef broth 2 Yukon gold potatoes, diced ¼ head cauliflower 1 (8 ounce) package shredded sharp Cheddar cheese

Directions and total time – 1-2 h • Turn on a multi-functional pressure cooker and select Saute function. Add turkey and seasoned salt; saute until browned, about 5 minutes. Remove turkey. • Melt butter in the pot. Add carrots, celery, and onion; cook until just starting to soften, about 5 minutes. Add flour, dill, and pepper; cook for about 1 minute. Return turkey to the pot; add broth and potatoes. Top with cauliflower. Close and lock the lid. • Select high pressure according to manufacturer's instructions; set timer for 10 minutes. Allow 10 to 15 minutes for pressure to build. • Release pressure carefully using the quick-release method according to manufacturer's instructions, about 5 minutes. Unlock and remove the lid. • Remove the cauliflower and 1 cup of the soup liquid; blend together until smooth and creamy. Add Cheddar cheese and season to tate. Stir cauliflower puree into the pot with the rest of the soup until cheese is completely melted.

Cabbage and Turkey Soup

Ingredients for 6 servings: 1 pound ground turkey ¼ cup diced onion ¼ cup diced green bell pepper ¼ cup diced celery ¼ cup diced carrot 2 teaspoons ground black pepper 1 teaspoon seasoned salt 1 teaspoon garlic salt 1 teaspoon garlic powder 1 teaspoon paprika 3 ½ cups chicken broth, or to taste 2 ½ cups chopped cabbage, or to taste 1 (14 ounce) can petite diced tomatoes 1 (8 ounce) can tomato sauce 1 tablespoon Worcestershire sauce 2 bay leaves ⅓ cup acini di pepe pasta

Directions and total time – 1-2 h • Turn on a multi-functional pressure cooker and select Saute function. Add ground turkey and cook, stirring, for about 5 minutes. Add onion, bell pepper, celery, carrot, black pepper, seasoned salt, garlic salt, garlic powder, and paprika; saute for another 5 minutes. • Add chicken broth, cabbage, diced tomatoes, tomato sauce, Worcestershire sauce, and bay leaves to the Instant Pot(R). Close and lock the lid. Select high pressure according to manufacturer's instructions; set timer for 16 minutes. Allow 10 minutes for pressure to build. •

Release pressure using the natural-release method according to manufacturer's instructions, about 5 minutes. Unlock and remove the lid. Add pasta; close and lock lid. Select high pressure according to manufacturer's instructions; set timer for 5 minutes. Allow 5 minutes for pressure to build. ● Release pressure using the natural-release method according to manufacturer's instructions, about 5 minutes.

Turkey Breast with Paprika

Ingredients for 8 servings:

4 lbs turkey breast boneless, thawed 1 tbsp olive oil 1 tbsp smoked paprika 1 tbsp italian seasoning 1 tsp tarragon 1 tsp salt 2 tsp pepper 2 cloves garlic minced 2 tbsp butter unsalted 2 tbsp olive oil For Gravy 2 tbsp butter unsalted 2 tbsp all-purpose flour ½ cup chicken broth ½ cup half and half

Directions and total time – 1 h

• Drizzle the tbsp of olive oil all over the turkey breast and rub it in. I usually do this so that the spices stick to the turkey breast. Rub the turkey well with the smoked paprika, Italian seasoning, tarragon, salt, and pepper. Finish with the minced garlic. • Turn the Instant Pot to the high saute setting. Add the 2 tbsp butter and oil and once your instant pot reaches the desired temperature (the timer will start to count down) add the turkey breast. Sear the turkey breast on all sides. Should take about 5 to 8 minutes.

Transfer the breast to a plate or a cutting board. • Add the Instant Pot's wire rack, then place the turkey on top, as seen in the video. Close the lid (follow the manufacturer's guide for instructions on how to close the instant pot lid). Set the Instant Pot to the Manual setting and set the timer to 25 minutes on high pressure. • Once the Instant Pot cycle is complete, wait until the natural release cycle is complete, should take about 10 to 15 minutes. Follow the manufacturer's guide for quick release, if in a rush. Carefully unlock and remove the lid from the instant pot. Transfer the breast to a cutting board, cover completely with aluminum foil and let it rest for 10 to 15 minutes before cutting into it. Make sure to remove the butcher twine before slicing it. If crispier skin is desired, broil it in the oven for an additional 5-10 minutes. For the Gravy: • Turn the Instant Pot to the high saute setting (don't discard the turkey drippings). Add the 2 tbsp of butter and cook until the butter is melted. Whisk in the flour with the butter and cook for a couple minutes, stirring or whisking constantly, until the flour loses its raw smell. • Whisk in the chicken broth and cook and half and half and cook for an additional 3 minutes or until thickened. You can omit the half and half and just use 1 cup of chicken broth or turkey broth. I used half and half for a creamier gravy. Season with salt and pepper as preferred.

Turkey-Stuffed Peppers

Ingredients for 4 servings:

4 large multicolored bell peppers, tops cut off and chopped, peppers hollowed and seeded 1 pound 93% lean ground turkey ¾ cup cooked brown rice [I love Trader Joe's frozen brown rice] ⅓ cup seasoned breadcrumbs ¾ cup reduced-sodium marinara sauce, divided ¼ cup minced onion 1 ounce grated Parmesan cheese (about ¼ cup) 3 tablespoons chopped parsley 2 teaspoons tomato paste ¼ teaspoon kosher salt Black pepper to taste 1 large egg, beaten 1 garlic clove, minced ½ cup water 1 ounce shredded mozzarella cheese (about ¼ cup)

Directions and total time – 30-60 m

• Step 1 Combine chopped pepper tops with ground turkey, cooked brown rice, breadcrumbs, ¼ cup marinara sauce, onion, Parmesan cheese, parsley, tomato paste, salt, black pepper, egg, and garlic. Mix thoroughly. • Step 2 Stuff about 1 cup ground turkey mixture into each pepper. Pour ½ cup water into bottom of Instant Pot. Place a rack in the pot; stand stuffed peppers upright on the rack. Cover each pepper top with 2 tablespoons marinara sauce. Cover and cook on high pressure 15 minutes; natural release. Open the lid, top with mozzarella cheese, and cover until cheese melts, about 2 minutes.

Turkey and Homemade Gravy

Ingredients for 8 servings:

Stock Ingredients for Cooking Pot: 2 Tablespoons Butter 2 teaspoons Kosher Salt 1 teaspoon Freshly Ground Black Pepper 1 large Yellow/Brown Onion quartered 2 stalks Fresh Celery 2 medium Carrots peeled and cut in half 4 cloves Fresh Garlic 1 inch Fresh Ginger Root peeled ½ teaspoon Peppercorns ¼ cup Dry White Wine or Marsala Wine ½ teaspoon Turkey Base (or vegetable base) 1 Bay Leaves 1 cup Fresh Water Turkey Preparation: 7 pound Bone In Turkey Breast with skin ¼ cup Potato Starch 1 Tablespoon Bells Turkey Seasoning 2 Tablespoons Butter Finishing: 2 Tablespoons All Purpose Flour (or Potato Starch)

Directions and total time – 30-60 m

• Pat dry Turkey. Massage seasonings into Turkey and then dredge through Potato Starch. Mix together Water and Turkey Base

(Bouillon) and set aside. • Select Sauté/Browning on Pressure Cooker and allow to fully heat. Add 2 Tablespoons Butter to cooking pot. Place Turkey Breast into cooking pot and brown the skin a bit. Carefully remove Breast from pot, making sure not to break off the Skin. • Pour ¼ cup Dry White Wine into cooking pot and deglaze pot to remove any bits that may have attached to the bottom of the pot. Add Broth and mix through, making sure to loosen all stuck on brown bits. • Once deglazed, place Carrots, Onions, Celery, Ginger, Peppercorns and Bay Leaf into cooking pot. • Shove a little Butter under the skin and place Turkey on Trivet, Breast side down. Lower into cooking pot and place the rest of the Butter in the cavity. • Lock on Lid and close Pressure Valve. Cook on LOW Pressure (most machines default to high) for 32 minutes. When Beep sounds, wait until all pressure has released naturally and then open the Lid. • Remove Turkey to a Serving Platter and cover. Strain Stock through a metal Strainer into a Bowl and discard solids. Use a Fat Separator to remove layer of fat, or skim from top. Place Stock back into cooking pot, reserving half a cup. • Select Sauté/Browning. Make a Slurry by adding 2 Tablespoons of Flour (or Potato Starch) to reserved Stock and Whisking until completely incorporated. Add Slurry to cooking pot and Whisk to incorporate. Simmer until desired consistency. • Mealthy CrispLid • If using the Mealthy Crisplid, add all the ingredients from the "For Cooking Pot" section to the cooking pot and then pick up with Instruction No. 5. • After pressure has released and the turkey is cooked, turn off Instant Pot and place the CripsLid on top of pot. Brush the turkey with a bit of olive oil. Set the temperature to 375 degrees and brown the turkey skin to your desired color. Remove turkey from pot and follow the gravy instructions.

Turkey Tenderloin

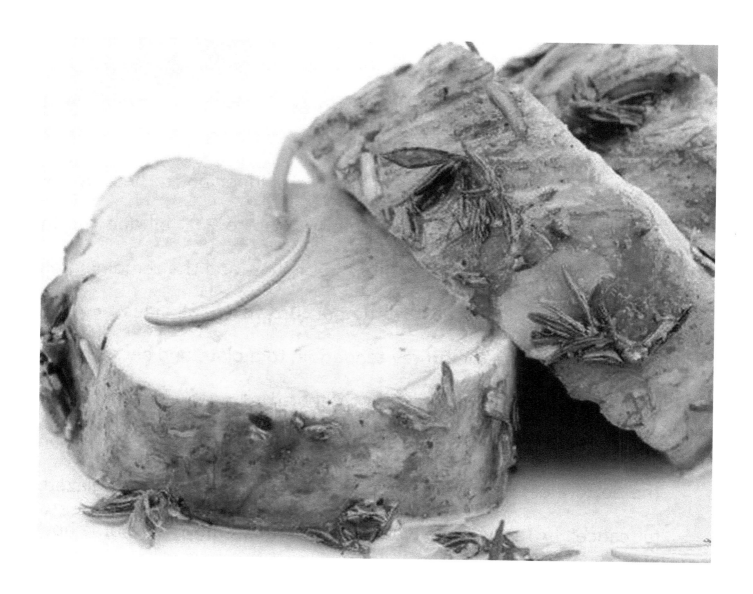

Ingredients for 4-6 servings:

1 Boneless Turkey Breast Tenderloin 4 T. Garlic Infused Oil 1 Medium Onion, cut into wedges 1 ½ c. Chicken Broth 1 t. Rosemary 1 t. Thyme 1. t. Oregano Salt and Pepper, to taste Cajun Rub, optional

Directions and total time – 30-60 m

• Turn Instant Pot on to sauté. Allow the inner pot to heat up. • Cover the turkey breast tenderloin with up to 2 T. oil and rub in the seasonings. • Once the inner pot is hot, add the remaining oil (2-3 T.) and turkey breast to the pot. Brown on all sides. • After browning, remove the turkey tenderloin to a plate and set aside. • Add 1 ½ c. of chicken broth to the pot. Use a wooden spatula to deglaze the bottom of the pot. Make sure all the browned bits on the bottom of the pot are scraped up. • Once the pot is deglazed, hit cancel. • Insert the trivet into the pot carefully (the pot is hot) and place the tenderloin on top of the trivet. Add in the onion wedges. • Place the lid on the pot and set the vent to sealing. • Pressure cook on "High/Manual" for 30 minutes. • Once the turkey is done cooking allow the pressure to release naturally.

Turkey with Drop Biscuit Dumplings

Ingredients for 8 servings:

Bones from a cooked bone-in turkey breast Trimmings from 1-2 leeks Trimmings from 3 carrots Trimmings from 3 celery stalks 1 teaspoon whole peppercorns 2 whole bay leaves 1 small sprig of fresh rosemary 5-6 sprigs of fresh thyme 2 whole garlic cloves 1 tablespoon apple cider vinegar Water For the stew: 1 teaspoon butter 2 teaspoons olive oil 1 ¼ cup small-diced carrots (about 3 medium carrots) 1 ¼ cup small-diced leeks (about 1 large or 2 small leeks) 1 ¼ cup small-diced celery (about 3 stalks) 1 teaspoon minced garlic 1 teaspoon finely chopped fresh thyme ½ teaspoon finely chopped fresh rosemary ¼ cup flour ½ cup white wine 5 cups turkey bone broth (from recipe above; or substitute with chicken or turkey stock) 4 cups shredded cooked turkey meat Salt and pepper to taste For the drop biscuits: 1 ¾ cups all-purpose flour (or 1 cup all-purpose and 1 cup white whole wheat) 2 teaspoons baking powder ½ teaspoon baking soda ½ teaspoon salt 4 tablespoons butter 1 cup cold low-fat buttermilk

Directions and total time – 1-2 h For the broth (optional):

• Place the bones of the turkey breast in the Instant Pot insert. Add the vegetable trimmings. Fill up to 1 inch below the max fill line with water. Add the peppercorns, bay leaves, fresh herbs, garlic, and cider vinegar. Place the lid on the Instant Pot and set to "sealing." Cook on high pressure for 45 minutes and allow for a 30-minute natural pressure release. • Carefully move the knob to "venting" and release any remainder of steam in the Instant Pot. Strain the broth through a fine-mesh strainer. Season to taste with salt. Cool completely before storing in the refrigerator. Remove 5 cups of broth for the dumpling stew. Chill the remainder and store in the fridge for when you reheat dumpling leftovers. For the stew: • Set the Instant Pot on "saute" mode. Add the butter and olive oil. Once the butter is melted, add the carrots, leeks, and celery. Saute until softened and translucent, about 5 minutes, being careful not to let anything burn on the bottom of the pot. Add the garlic, thyme, and rosemary, stirring until fragrant, about 30 seconds. Add the flour and stir to coat the vegetables. Add the wine to deglaze, scraping up any bits on the bottom and sides of the pot. Add the broth and shredded turkey, stirring until the mixture comes to a simmer, about 4 minutes. Press "cancel" on the Instant Pot to turn off the heat. Season to taste with salt and pepper. Remove the pot insert from the Instant Pot while you make the dumplings to ensure that nothing sticks to the bottom and the sides. • For the dumplings: • In a medium bowl, combine the flour, salt, baking powder, and baking soda. Melt the butter, and after cooling for 2-3 minutes, add it to the buttermilk. Let it stand in the buttermilk for 2-3 minutes. Stir the mixture together until the butter forms clumps in the buttermilk. Add this mixture to the flour mixture and use a rubber spatula to stir it into the flour until just combined. Use a small cookie dough scoop to scoop the drop biscuits into the turkey mixture in the Instant Pot insert. You should have 18-20 dumplings total. • Return the insert to the Instant Pot and place the lid on top. Set the knob to "sealing." Cook on high pressure for 3 minutes. Carefully quick release the pressure manually, allowing all the steam to escape. Ladle the stew and dumplings into bowls and serve warm! • Reheat leftovers and add extra turkey broth as needed to get the desired consistency you like as you reheat. • Note: if for some reason you get "burn" notice on the Instant Pot, no worries! Just release the pressure, remove the lid, and turn the Instant Pot to "saute" mode. Bring the mixture to a simmer and cook the dumplings, carefully stirring often with a rubber spatula, for 5 minutes. Ladle into bowls and serve. Stovetop instructions: • Place a large pot over medium heat. Add the butter and olive oil. Once the butter is melted, add the carrots, leeks, and celery. Saute for 5-6 minutes until softened and translucent. Add the garlic, thyme, and rosemary, stirring until fragrant, about 30 seconds. Add the flour and stir to coat the vegetables. Add the wine to deglaze, scraping up any bits on the bottom and sides of the pot. Add the broth and shredded turkey, stirring until the mixture comes to a simmer, about 4-5 minutes. • Use a small cookie dough scoop to scoop the drop biscuits into the turkey mixture. You should have 18-20 dumplings total. Place the lid on the pot and simmer over low heat for 10 minutes. Remove lid and serve

Apple Pie Granola

(Ready in about 1 hour 35 minutes | Servings 4)

Per serving: 234 Calories; 22.2g Fat; 9.5g Carbs; 2.5g Protein; 5.3g Sugars

Ingredients

3 tablespoons coconut oil 1 teaspoon stevia powder 1 cup coconut, shredded 1/4 cup walnuts, chopped 1 ½ tablespoons sunflower seeds 1 ½ tablespoons pumpkin seeds 1 teaspoon apple pie spice mix A pinch of salt 1 small apple, sliced

Directions Place coconut oil, stevia powder, coconut, walnuts, sunflower seeds, pumpkin seeds, apple pie spice mix, and salt in your Instant Pot. Secure the lid. Choose "Slow Cook" mode and High pressure; cook for 1 hours 30 minutes. Once cooking is complete, use a quick pressure release; carefully remove the lid.

Spoon into individual bowls, garnish with apples and serve warm.

Bon appétit!

Shirred Eggs with Peppers and Scallions

(Ready in about 10 minutes | Servings 4)

Per serving: 208 Calories; 18.7g Fat; 3.9g Carbs; 6.7g Protein; 2.3g Sugars

Ingredients

4 tablespoons butter, melted 4 tablespoons double cream 4 eggs 4 scallions, chopped 2 red peppers, seeded and chopped 1/2 teaspoon granulated garlic 1/4 teaspoon dill weed 1/4 teaspoon sea salt 1/4 teaspoon freshly ground pepper

Directions

Start by adding 1 cup of water and a metal rack to the Instant Pot. Grease the bottom and sides of each ramekin with melted butter. Divide the ingredients among the prepared four ramekins. Lower the ramekins onto the metal rack. Secure the lid. Choose "Manual" mode and High pressure; cook for 5 minutes. Once cooking is complete, use a natural pressure release; carefully remove the lid.

Bon appétit!

Breakfast Meatloaf Cups

(Ready in about 40 minutes | Servings 8)

Per serving: 375 Calories; 22.2g Fat; 6.5g Carbs; 35.4g Protein; 4.5g Sugars

Ingredients

1 pound ground pork 1 pound ground beef 1/2 cup onion, chopped 2 garlic cloves, minced Salt and ground black pepper, to taste 1/3 cup Romano cheese, grated 1/4 cup pork rinds, crushed 4 eggs, whisked 2 ripe tomatoes, puréed 1/4 cup barbecue sauce, sugar-free

Directions

Start by adding 1 cup of water and a metal trivet to the bottom of your Instant Pot. In a mixing bowl, thoroughly combine ground meat, onion, garlic, salt, black pepper, cheese, pork rinds, and eggs. Mix until everything is well incorporated. Divide the mixture among muffin cups. In a small mixing bowl, whisk puréed tomatoes with barbecue sauce. Lastly, top your muffins with the tomato sauce. Secure the lid. Choose "Manual" mode and High pressure; cook for 25 minutes. Once cooking is complete, use a quick pressure release; carefully remove the lid. Allow them to cool for 10 minutes before removing from the muffin tin. Bon appétit!

Spicy and Cheesy Chard Quiche

(Ready in about 35 minutes | Servings 6)

Per serving: 183 Calories; 14.4g Fat; 5.6g Carbs; 8.1g Protein; 2.8g Sugars

Ingredients

10 large eggs 1/2 cup double cream Seasoned salt and ground black pepper, to taste 1 teaspoon cayenne pepper 2 cups chard, roughly chopped 1 habanero pepper, seeded and chopped 1 tomato, chopped 1/2 cup red onion, thinly sliced 1/2 cup Pepper-Jack cheese, freshly grated

Directions

Start by adding 1 ½ cups of water and a metal trivet to the bottom of your Instant Pot. Now, lightly grease a baking dish with a nonstick cooking spray. In a mixing bowl, thoroughly combine the eggs with double cream, salt, black pepper, and cayenne pepper.

Now, stir in the chard, habanero pepper, tomato, and onion. Spoon the mixture into the prepared baking dish. Cover with a piece of aluminum foil, making a foil sling. Secure the lid. Choose "Manual" mode and High pressure; cook for 20 minutes. Once cooking is complete, use a quick pressure release; carefully remove the lid. Top with cheese and cover with the lid; allow it to sit in the residual heat for 10 minutes. Serve immediately and enjoy!

Hungarian Hot Pot

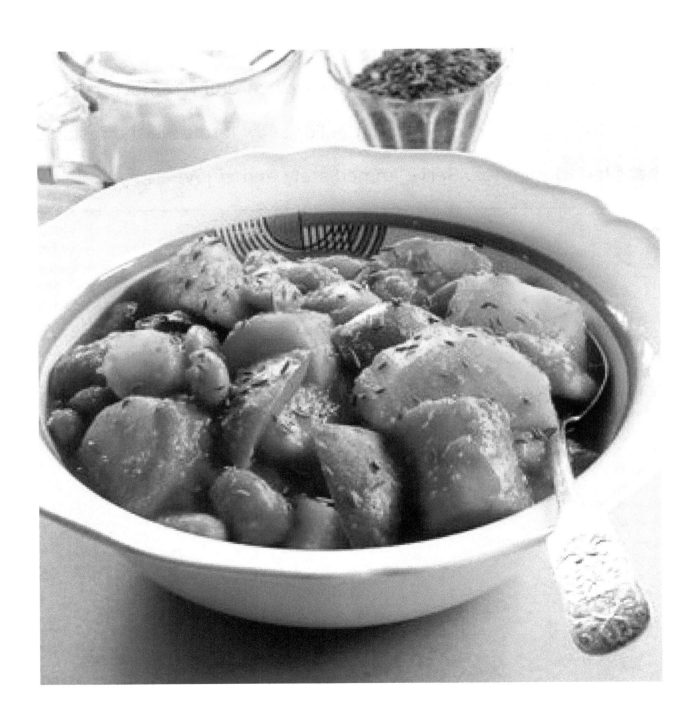

(Ready in about 15 minutes | Servings 4)

Per serving: 292 Calories; 21.6g Fat; 8.4g Carbs; 15.7g Protein; 3.5g Sugars

Ingredients

1 tablespoon grapeseed oil 9 ounces Hungarian smoked sausage, casing removed and sliced 1 carrot, cut into thick slices 1 celery stalk, diced 2 bell peppers, cut into wedges 2 cups roasted vegetable broth 1/2 cup shallot, peeled and diced Sea salt and ground black pepper, to taste 1/2 tablespoon hot pepper flakes 1 bay leaf 1/4 cup fresh cilantro leaves, roughly chopped

Directions

Press the "Sauté" button to heat up the Instant Pot. Now, heat the oil and brown the sausage for 2 to 3 minutes. Stir in the other ingredients. Secure the lid. Choose "Manual" mode and High pressure; cook for 10 minutes. Once cooking is complete, use a

natural pressure release; carefully remove the lid. Bon appétit!

Dilled Cauliflower Purée with Au Jus Gravy

(Ready in about 20 minutes | Servings 4)

Per serving: 291 Calories; 26.6g Fat; 8.1g Carbs; 7.1g Protein; 4.5g Sugars

Ingredients

Cauliflower Purée: 1 head of fresh cauliflower, broken into florets 1/4 cup double cream 2 tablespoons butter 3 cloves garlic minced 4 tablespoons Romano cheese, grated 1 teaspoon dried dill weed Kosher salt and ground black pepper, to taste Gravy: 1 ½ cups beef stock 1/2 cup double cream 3 tablespoons butter

Directions

Add 1 cup of water and a steamer basket to the bottom of your Instant Pot. Then, arrange cauliflower in the steamer basket. Secure the lid. Choose "Manual" mode and Low pressure; cook for 3 minutes. Once cooking is complete, use a quick pressure release;

carefully remove the lid. Now, puree the cauliflower with a potato masher. Add the remaining ingredients for the purée and stir well. Press the "Sauté" button to heat up the Instant Pot. Now, combine the ingredients for the gravy and let it simmer for 10 minutes. Stir until the gravy thickens down to a consistency of your liking. Serve cauliflower purée with the gravy on the side. Bon appétit!

Coconut Porridge with Berries

(Ready in about 10 minutes | Servings 2)

Per serving: 242 Calories; 20.7g Fat; 7.9g Carbs; 7.6g Protein; 2.8g Sugars

Ingredients

4 tablespoons coconut flour 1 tablespoon sunflower seeds 3 tablespoons flax meal 1 ¼ cups water 1/4 teaspoon coarse salt 1/4 teaspoon grated nutmeg 1/2 teaspoon ground cardamom 2 eggs, beaten 2 tablespoons coconut oil, softened 2 tablespoons Swerve 1/2 cup mixed berries, fresh or frozen (thawed)

Directions

Add all ingredients, except for mixed berries, to the Instant Pot. Secure the lid. Choose "Manual" mode and High pressure; cook for 5 minutes. Once cooking is complete, use a quick pressure release;

carefully remove the lid. Divide between two bowls, top with berries, and serve hot. Bon appétit!

Zucchini Sloppy Joe's

(Ready in about 10 minutes | Servings 2

Per serving: 159 Calories; 9.8g Fat; 1.5g Carbs; 15.5g Protein; 0.7g Sugars

Ingredients

1 tablespoon olive oil 1/2 pound ground beef Salt and ground black pepper, to taste 1 medium-sized zucchini, cut into 4 slices lengthwise 1 tomato, sliced 4 lettuce leaves 2 teaspoons mustard

Directions

Add olive oil, ground beef, salt, and black pepper to your Instant Pot. Secure the lid. Choose "Manual" mode and High pressure; cook for 5 minutes. Once cooking is complete, use a natural pressure release; carefully remove the lid. Divide the ground meat mixture between 2 zucchini slices. Add tomato slices, lettuce, and mustard. Top with the second slice of zucchini. Bon appétit!

Fluffy Berry Cupcakes

(Ready in about 30 minutes | Servings 6)

Per serving: 238 Calories; 21.6g Fat; 4.1g Carbs; 7.5g Protein; 2.2g Sugars

Ingredients

1/4 cup coconut oil, softened 3 ounces cream cheese, softened 1/4 cup double cream 4 eggs 1/4 cup coconut flour 1/4 cup almond flour A pinch of salt 1/3 cup Swerve, granulated 1 teaspoon baking powder 1/4 teaspoon cardamom powder 1/2 teaspoon star anise, ground 1/2 cup fresh mixed berries

Directions

Start by adding 1 ½ cups of water and a metal rack to your Instant Pot. Mix coconut oil, cream cheese, and double cream in a bowl. Fold in the eggs, one at a time, and continue to mix until everything is well incorporated. In another bowl, thoroughly combine the flour, salt, Swerve, baking powder, cardamom, and anise. Add the cream/egg mixture to this dry mixture. Afterwards, fold in fresh berries and gently stir to combine. Divide the batter between silicone cupcake liners. Cover with a piece of foil. Place the cupcakes on the rack. Secure the lid. Choose "Manual" mode and High pressure; cook for 25 minutes. Once cooking is complete, use a natural pressure release; carefully remove the lid. Enjoy!

Salmon and Ricotta Fat Bombs

(Ready in about 15 minutes | Servings 6)

Per serving: 130 Calories; 9.1g Fat; 1.7g Carbs; 10.2g Protein; 0.5g Sugars

Ingredients

1/2 pound salmon fillets Salt and ground black pepper, to taste 1/4 teaspoon smoked paprika 1/4 teaspoon hot paprika 2 tablespoons butter, softened 4 ounces Ricotta cheese, room temperature 1/4 cup green onions, chopped 1 garlic clove, finely chopped 2 teaspoons fresh parsley, finely chopped

Directions

Start by adding 1 ½ cups of water and a metal rack to the bottom of your Instant Pot. Place the salmon on the metal rack. Secure the lid. Choose "Manual" mode and Low pressure; cook for 8 minutes. Once cooking is complete, use a quick pressure release; carefully remove the lid. Chop the salmon. Add the salt, pepper, paprika, butter, cheese, onions, and garlic. Shape the mixture into balls and roll them in chopped parsley. Arrange fat bombs on a serving platter and enjoy!

Greek-Style Mushroom Muffins

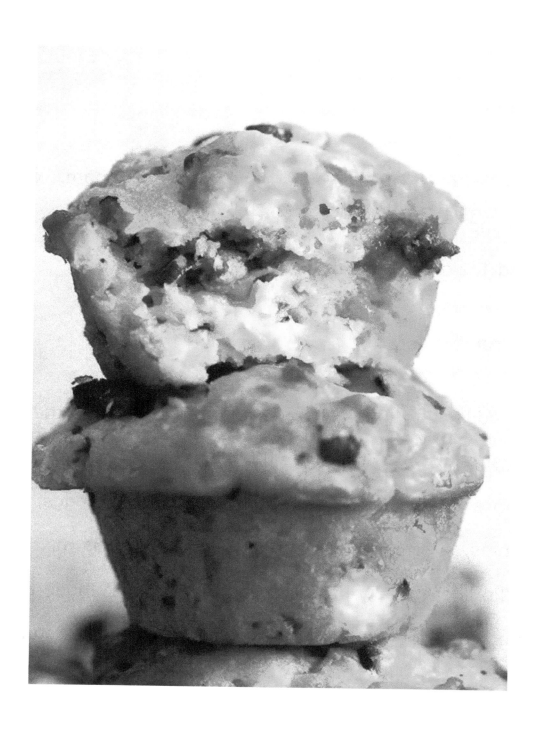

(Ready in about 10 minutes | Servings 6)

Per serving: 259 Calories; 18.9g Fat; 6.7g Carbs; 15.7g Protein; 3.9g Sugars

Ingredients

6 eggs 1 red onion, chopped 2 cups button mushrooms, chopped Sea salt and ground black pepper, to taste 1 ½ cups Feta cheese, shredded 1/2 cup Kalamata olives, pitted and sliced

Directions

Start by adding 1 ½ cups of water and a metal rack to the bottom of the Instant Pot. Spritz each muffin liner with a nonstick cooking spray. In a mixing bowl, thoroughly combine the eggs, onions, mushrooms, salt, and black pepper. Now, pour this mixture into the muffin liners. Secure the lid. Choose "Manual" mode and Low pressure; cook for 7 minutes. Once cooking is complete, use a quick pressure release; carefully remove the lid. Sprinkle cheese and olives on top of the cups; cover with the lid for a few minutes to allow it to melt. Enjoy!

Easy Spinach Dip

(Ready in about 5 minutes | Servings 10)

Per serving: 43 Calories; 1.7g Fat; 3.5g Carbs; 4.1g Protein; 1.3g Sugars

Ingredients

1 pound spinach 4 ounces Cottage cheese, at room temperature 4 ounces Cheddar cheese, grated 1 teaspoon garlic powder 1/2 teaspoon shallot powder 1/2 teaspoon celery seeds 1/2 teaspoon fennel seeds 1/2 teaspoon cayenne pepper Salt and black pepper, to taste

Directions

Add all of the above ingredients to your Instant Pot. Secure the lid. Choose "Manual" mode and High pressure; cook for 1 minute. Once cooking is complete, use a quick pressure release; carefully remove the lid. Serve warm or at room temperature. Bon appétit!

Cheesy Mustard Greens Dip

(Ready in about 10 minutes | Servings 10)

Per serving: 153 Calories; 10.6g Fat; 7g Carbs; 8.7g Protein; 3.6g Sugars

Ingredients

2 tablespoons butter, melted 20 ounces mustard greens 2 bell peppers, chopped 1 white onion, chopped 1 teaspoon garlic, minced Sea salt and ground black pepper, to taste 1 cup chicken stock 8 ounces Neufchâtel cheese, crumbled 1/2 teaspoon dried thyme 1/2 teaspoon dried dill 1/2 teaspoon turmeric powder 3/4 cup Romano cheese, preferably freshly grated

Directions

Add the butter, mustard greens, bell peppers, onion, and garlic to the Instant Pot. Secure the lid. Choose "Manual" mode and High pressure; cook for 3 minutes. Once cooking is complete, use a quick pressure release; carefully remove the lid. Then, add the remaining ingredients and press the "Sauté" button. Let it simmer until the cheese is melted; then, gently stir this mixture until everything is well incorporated. Serve with your favorite low-carb dippers.

Colorful Stuffed Mushrooms

(Ready in about 10 minutes | Servings 5)

Per serving: 151 Calories; 9.2g Fat; 6g Carbs; 11.9g Protein; 3.6g Sugars

Ingredients

1 tablespoon butter, softened 1 shallot, chopped 2 cloves garlic, minced 1 ½ cups Cottage cheese, at room temperature 1/2 cup Romano cheese, grated 1 red bell pepper, chopped 1 green bell pepper, chopped 1 jalapeno pepper, minced 1/2 teaspoon dried basil 1/2 teaspoon dried oregano 1/2 teaspoon dried rosemary 10 medium-sized button mushrooms, stems removed

Directions

Press the "Sauté" button to heat up your Instant Pot. Once hot, melt the butter and sauté the shallots until tender and translucent. Stir in the garlic and cook an additional 30 seconds or until aromatic. Now, add the remaining ingredients, except for the mushroom caps, and stir to combine well. Then, fill the mushroom caps with this mixture. Add 1 cup of water and a steamer basket to you Instant Pot. Arrange the stuffed mushrooms in the steamer basket. Secure the lid. Choose "Manual" mode and High pressure; cook for 5 minutes. Once cooking is complete, use a quick pressure release; carefully remove the lid. Arrange the stuffed mushroom on a serving platter and serve. Enjoy!

Herbed and Caramelized Mushrooms

(Ready in about 10 minutes | Servings 4)

Per serving: 91 Calories; 6.4g Fat; 5.5g Carbs; 5.2g Protein; 2.8g Sugars

Ingredients

2 tablespoons butter, melted 20 ounces button mushrooms, brushed clean 2 cloves garlic, minced 1 teaspoon dried basil 1 teaspoon dried rosemary 1 teaspoon dried sage 1 bay leaf Sea salt, to taste 1/2 teaspoon freshly ground black pepper 1/2 cup water 1/2 cup broth, preferably homemade 1 tablespoon soy sauce 1 tablespoon fresh parsley leaves, roughly chopped

Directions

Press the "Sauté" button to heat up your Instant Pot. Once hot, melt the butter and sauté the mushrooms and garlic until aromatic. Add seasonings, water, and broth. Add garlic, oregano, mushrooms, thyme, basil, bay leaves, veggie broth, and salt and pepper to your instant pot. Secure the lid. Choose "Manual" mode and High pressure; cook for 5 minutes. Once cooking is complete, use a quick pressure release; carefully remove the lid. Arrange your mushrooms on a serving platter and serve with cocktail sticks. Bon appétit!

Party Chicken Drumettes

(Ready in about 15 minutes | Servings 8)

Per serving: 237 Calories; 20.6g Fat; 3.1g Carbs; 10.2g Protein; 1.8g Sugars

Ingredients

2 pounds chicken drumettes 1 stick butter 1 tablespoon coconut aminos Sea salt and ground black pepper, to taste 1/2 teaspoon dried dill weed 1/2 teaspoon dried basil 1 teaspoon hot sauce 1 tablespoon fish sauce 1/2 cup tomato sauce 1/2 cup water

Directions

Add all ingredients to your Instant Pot. Secure the lid. Choose "Poultry" mode and High pressure; cook for 10 minutes. Once cooking is complete, use a natural pressure release; carefully remove the lid. Serve at room temperature and enjoy!

Crave-Worthy Balsamic Baby Carrots

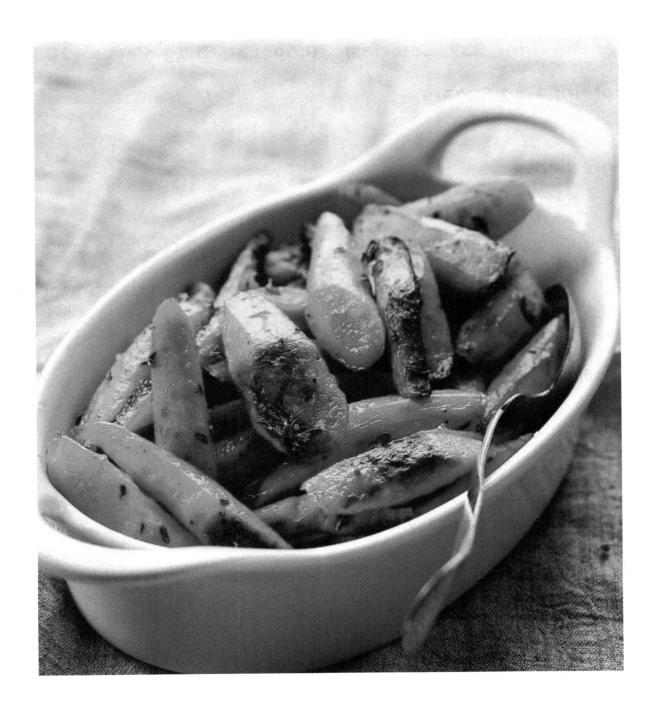

(Ready in about 10 minutes | Servings 8)

Per serving: 94 Calories; 6.1g Fat; 8.9g Carbs; 1.4g Protein; 4.1g Sugars

Ingredients

28 ounces baby carrots 1 cup chicken broth 1/2 cup water 1/2 stick butter 2 tablespoons balsamic vinegar Coarse sea salt, to taste 1/2 teaspoon red pepper flakes, crushed 1/2 teaspoon dried dill weed

Directions

Simply add all of the above ingredients to your Instant Pot. Secure the lid. Choose "Manual" mode and High pressure; cook for 3 minutes. Once cooking is complete, use a quick pressure release; carefully remove the lid. Transfer to a nice serving bowl and serve. Enjoy!

___

Minty Party Meatballs

(Ready in about 15 minutes | Servings 6)

Per serving: 280 Calories; 20.4g Fat; 3.7g Carbs; 20.6g Protein; 2.5g Sugars

Ingredients

1/2 pound ground pork 1/2 pound ground turkey 2 eggs 1/3 cup almond flour Sea salt and ground black pepper, to taste 2 garlic cloves, minced 1 cup Romano cheese, grated 1 teaspoon dried basil 1/2 teaspoon dried thyme 1/4 cup minced fresh mint, plus more for garnish 1/2 cup beef bone broth 1/2 cup tomatoes, puréed 2 tablespoons scallions

Directions

Thoroughly combine all ingredients, except for broth, tomatoes, and scallions in a mixing bowl. Shape the mixture into 2-inch meatballs and reserve. Add beef bone broth, tomatoes, and scallions to your Instant Pot. Place the meatballs in this sauce. Secure the lid. Choose "Manual" mode and High pressure; cook for 8 minutes. Once cooking is complete, use a quick pressure release; carefully remove the lid. Bon appétit!

Amazing Cauliflower Tots

(Ready in about 25 minutes | Servings 6)

Per serving: 132 Calories; 8.7g Fat; 4.5g Carbs; 9.2g Protein; 1.3g Sugars

Ingredients

1 head of cauliflower, broken into florets 2 eggs, beaten 1 shallot, peeled and chopped 1/2 cup Swiss cheese, grated 1/2 cup Parmesan cheese, grated 2 tablespoons fresh coriander, chopped Sea salt and ground black pepper, to taste

Directions

Start by adding 1 cup of water and a steamer basket to your Instant Pot. Arrange the cauliflower florets in the steamer basket. Secure the lid. Choose "Manual" mode and High pressure; cook for 3 minutes. Once cooking is complete, use a quick pressure release; carefully remove the lid. Mash the cauliflower and add the remaining ingredients. Form the mixture into a tater-tot shape with oiled hands. Place cauliflower tots on a lightly greased baking sheet. Bake in the preheated oven at 390 degrees F approximately 20 minutes; make sure to flip them halfway through the cooking time. Serve at room temperature. Bon appétit!

Gruyère, Rutabaga and Bacon Bites

(Ready in about 10 minutes | Servings 8)

Per serving: 187 Calories; 14.2g Fat; 5.2g Carbs; 9.4g Protein; 3.4g Sugars

Ingredients

1/2 pound rutabaga, grated 4 slices meaty bacon, chopped 7 ounces Gruyère cheese, shredded 3 eggs, beaten 3 tablespoons almond flour 1 teaspoon granulated garlic 1 teaspoon shallot powder Sea salt and ground black pepper, to taste

Directions

Add 1 cup of water and a metal trivet to the Instant Pot. Mix all of the above ingredients until everything is well incorporated. Put the mixture into a silicone pod tray that is previously greased with a nonstick cooking spray. Cover the tray with a sheet of aluminum foil and lower it onto the trivet. Secure the lid. Choose "Manual" mode and Low pressure; cook for 5 minutes. Once cooking is complete, use a quick pressure release; carefully remove the lid. Bon appétit!

Spring Deviled Eggs

(Ready in about 25 minutes | Servings 8)

Per serving: 158 Calories; 12.1g Fat; 2.1g Carbs; 9.5g Protein; 1.2g Sugars

Ingredients

8 eggs Salt and white pepper, to taste 1/4 cup mayonnaise 1/2 can tuna in spring water, drained 2 tablespoons spring onions, finely chopped 1 teaspoon smoked cayenne pepper 1/3 teaspoon fresh or dried dill weed 1 teaspoon Dijon mustard 1 pickled jalapeño, minced

Directions

Place 1 cup of water and a steamer basket in your Instant Pot. Now, arrange the eggs on the steamer basket. Secure the lid. Choose "Manual" mode and Low pressure; cook for 5 minutes. Once cooking is complete, use a quick pressure release; carefully remove the lid. Allow the eggs to cool for 15 minutes. Peel the eggs and slice them into halves. Smash the egg yolks with a fork and add the remaining ingredients. Stir to combine well. Afterwards, stuff the egg whites with tuna mixture. Serve well-chilled and enjoy!

Cheese-Stuffed Cocktail Meatballs

(Ready in about 15 minutes | Servings 8)

Per serving: 277 Calories; 17.4g Fat; 3.1g Carbs; 25.8g Protein; 0.9g Sugars

Ingredients

1 pound ground beef 1/2 cup pork chicharron, crushed 1/2 cup Parmesan cheese, grated 2 eggs, beaten 2 tablespoons fresh scallions, chopped 2 tablespoons fresh cilantro, chopped 1 teaspoon garlic, minced Sea salt, to your liking 1/2 teaspoon ground black pepper 1/2 teaspoon cayenne pepper 1 cup Colby cheese, cubed 2 teaspoons olive oil 1/2 cup chicken broth 1/2 cup BBQ sauce

Directions

In a mixing dish, thoroughly combine ground beef, pork chicharron, Parmesan cheese, eggs, scallions, cilantro, garlic, salt, black pepper, and cayenne pepper; mix until everything is well incorporated. Now, shape the mixture into balls. Press one cheese cube into center of each meatball, sealing it inside. Press the "Sauté" button and heat the olive oil. Sear the meatballs for a couple of minutes or until browned on all sides. Pour in chicken broth and BBQ sauce. Secure the lid. Choose the "Manual" setting and cook for 8 minutes under High pressure. Once cooking is complete, use a quick pressure release; carefully remove the lid. Serve your meatballs with the sauce. Bon appétit!

Bacon Wrapped Cocktail Wieners

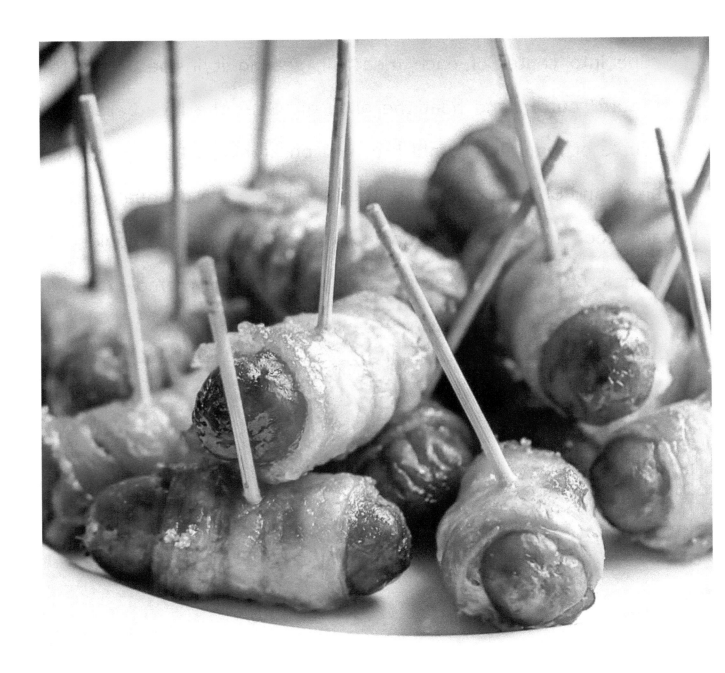

(Ready in about 10 minutes | Servings 10)

Per serving: 257 Calories; 22.7g Fat; 1.4g Carbs; 10.8g Protein; 0.2g Sugars

Ingredients

1 pound cocktail wieners 1/2 pound sliced bacon, cold cut into slices 1/2 cup chicken broth 1/2 cup water 1/4 cup low-carb ketchup 2 tablespoons apple cider vinegar 1 tablespoon onion powder 1 tablespoon ground mustard Salt and pepper to taste

Directions

Wrap each cocktail wiener with a slice of bacon; secure with a toothpick. Then, place one layer of bacon wrapped cocktail wieners in the bottom of the Instant Pot. Repeat layering until you run out of the cocktail wieners. In a mixing bowl, thoroughly combine the remaining ingredients. Pour this mixture over the bacon wrapped cocktail wieners. Secure the lid. Choose "Manual" mode and Low pressure; cook for 3 minutes. Once cooking is complete, use a natural pressure release; carefully remove the lid. Enjoy!

CPSIA information can be obtained
at www.ICGtesting.com
Printed in the USA
LVHW020910270521
688665LV00019B/1180